Heart Healthy Power Cocktails™

101 Recipes

By

Peter L. Johnston

ISBN-13: 978-1514793015

ISBN-10: 1514793016

DEDICATION

This book is dedicated to everyone who strives to rid the world of heart disease. One day, we will achieve this important goal.

CONTENTS

Introduction

Congratulations for taking the next step to becoming more heart healthy and welcome to our Heart healthy Power Cocktails™ Program! You are now in a group of countless others who use this program to become more heart healthy.

The chore of only eating heart healthy food is not always feasible for most people. However, having one or more Heart Healthy Power Cocktails™ a day is easy, healthy and fun! All of the 101 cocktails in the recipe chapter contain (only) nutrients that researchers have proven to help build a healthy heart. Even the herbs and spices are beneficial for building a healthy heart. So, each Power Cocktail™ packs a huge nutrient punch to improve your heart and cardio vascular system.

How to Use the Recipes

The recipes in this book were formulated by using ONLY ingredients that are healthy for the heart and cardio vascular system. The combination of ingredients in each drink recipe was based on taste, so that each of the recipes is pleasant to drink. The portions used in each recipe were determined for overall taste. Therefore, you can safely change the portioning to fit your taste, if you desire. In other words, you might choose to add more or less of apple juice to a particular drink. This is fine and encouraged. Experiment with each of the recipes and modify them to your liking. Then, you'll be more likely to drink them more often!

Adding Water. All of the recipes will need water added to them, usually at least a ½ of a cup. We decided to leave 'water' off of the ingredients listings because each person prefers a different consistency for their drinks. Therefore, when you blend the ingredients, we recommend starting the blending after adding ½ cup of water. After the drink is blended, if the mixture is too thick for your preference, add ¼ cup more water and blend again. Keep adding small portions of water until the mixture is the right consistency and taste for your preference.

To Juice or Not To Juice? You can juice the drinks in a juicer or blend them in a blender. However, we highly recommend that you blend the drinks so that you get the added benefits of more fiber in your diet. Unfortunately, a juicing machine removes fiber. Many doctors agree that adding more fiber to one's diet is the single-most important thing you can do to help build a healthy heart. So, do your heart a favor and blend your Power Cocktails instead of juicing.

Should I Steam, Cook or Blend the Vegetables in their Raw Form? Using raw vegetables is always preferred, as some nutrients are lost during cooking. However, some ingredients like raw sweet potatoes will not blend very well. Steam (preferred) or gently cook the vegetables in a small amount of water if you don't use raw vegetables. Do not overcook; only cook them long enough to soften them up. After you cook the vegetables, retain the left over water in the pan, since this water contains many of the lost nutrients. Then, add this left-over water to your mixture before blending, starting off with a ½ of a cup, and later adding more if you desire a thinner consistency.

Should I Make Individual Drinks or Batches? You can make single serving drinks, but it's easier to make a large batch of a recipe and refrigerate it for continued use. Each prepared cocktail is good for three days in a refrigerator. If you freeze a large batch, it will be good for at least 6 months. Many people prepare two different recipes at once, store them in the refrigerator, and then rotate drinking between the two recipes until the cocktails are gone. Then, they prepare two more batches of different recipes. In this manner, they keep from getting bored with the same drink.

How Many Cocktails Should I Drink Every Day? You should always seek the advice of your health care provider before making any major changes to your diet. However, these cocktails are made from real healthy heart food. None of the recipes contain vitamins or supplements in concentrated forms. So, it's not much different from including heart healthy foods on your dinner plate… the cocktails are just blended together for better taste and convenience. Many people drink one or two of these cocktails consistently every day. We also recommend that you drink a variety of the Power Cocktails™ so that you benefit from a wider variety of nutrients. In other words, don't just drink the Power Cocktails™ that contain dark chocolate!

Preparing Vegetables and Fruits. Some of the vegetables will need a little extra preparation before they are blended, especially foods like apples, oranges, and melons that contain non-edible seeds or rinds. The general rule of thumb is, "If you wouldn't normally eat that seed or rind, don't put it in your blended drink!' It's also a good idea to manually chop the fruits and vegetables so that they will blend easily without damaging your blender. For example, you might want to cut apples into eight sections before placing them in your blender.

Recipes

1 – Morning Wake-up Juice

1 cup of prepared green tea (can be replaced with black tea)
3 carrots
1 apple
1 orange

2 – Spicy Orange Sunshine

1 apple
1 orange
¼ teaspoon of cinnamon

3 – Southwest Cocktail

1 cup of black or kidney beans
2 cups of tomatoes
1 cup of water

4 – Sweet Sensations

3 carrots
1 cup of sweet potatoes
¼ teaspoon of cinnamon

5- Goody Juice

1 cup of spinach
1 cup of broccoli
1 cup of tomatoes

6 – Hearty Juice

2 cup of tomatoes
1 cup of red bell peppers
1 cup of steamed asparagus
¼ teaspoon of black pepper

7- Protein Plus-up

1 cup tofu
2 cups of tomatoes

8- Sweet Pastures

1 cup of acorn squash
1 cup of sweet potatoes
¼ teaspoon of sage

9- Chocolate milk

1 cup soy or almond milk
½ cup of dark chocolate

10- Sweet Potato Cocktail

1 cup of sweet potatoes
3 carrots
1 cup of tofu

11- Healthy Skyway

1 cup of tomatoes
3 carrots
1 cup of spinach
½ cup of broccoli
½ teaspoon of basil

12- Asian Mist Cocktail

1 cup of brown rice
3 cup of tomatoes
½ cup of black or kidney beans

13- Garden Treat

1 cup of cabbage
4 carrots
2 cups of tomatoes

14- Blueberry Pick-me-up

1 cup of prepared green or black tea
1/2 cup of blueberries (can be substituted with any type of berry)

15- Delightful Daze

1 cup of red bell peppers
1 cup of asparagus
1 cup of spinach
¼ teaspoon of black pepper

16- Garden Salad Juice

1 cup of lettuce
1 cup of spinach
1 cup of broccoli
3 carrots
1 teaspoon of olive oil

17-Pepper Asparagus Juice

2 cups of tomatoes
1 cup of asparagus
1 dash of black pepper

18 – Tomato-mato

1/2 cup of tofu
2 cups of tomatoes
1 dash of black pepper

19- Taste Bud Delight

5 carrots
1 stalk of celery
1 cup of apples
1 cup of Broccoli
½ cup of asparagus
1 tablespoon of olive oil

20- Breezy Asparagus

6 carrots
1 stalk of celery
½ cup of asparagus

21- Beet Treat

4 carrots
1 beet
1 Apple
1 Celery stalk
1 cup of spinach

22- Sassy Sally Juice

1 beet
4 carrots
½ cup of orange
1 cup of spinach
1 tablespoon of lemon or lime juice

23- Innocent Surprise

1 apple
1 celery stalk
1 orange
1 cup of sweet potatoes

24- Beet This!

6 carrots
2 cups of beets
1 cup of sweet potatoes

25- Easy Tomato Juice

1 cup of tomatoes
1 celery stalk
½ cup of red peppers

26- Special Tuna Surprise

1 can of tuna (drained)
1 cup of tomatoes
1 cup of red bell peppers
1 tablespoon of olive oil
¼ teaspoon of black pepper

27- Tuna Salad Cocktail

1 can of tuna (drained)
1 cup of tomatoes
2 carrots
1 cup of spinach
1 cup of broccoli

28- Protein-Plus Juice

1 cup of black or kidney beans
1 cup of tofu
2 cups of tomatoes

29- Zesty Tofu Cocktail

1 cup of tofu
5 carrots
1 cup of sweet potatoes
1 teaspoon of olive oil

30- Healing Melody

5 carrots
1 apple
1 stalk of celery

31- Grand Veggies Juice

1 cup of any dark green vegetable
2 cups of tomatoes
1 stalk of celery
1 dash of black pepper

32- Grandma's Apple Orchard Juice

1 cup of oatmeal (cooked or uncooked)
3 cup of apples

33- Southern Spells

1 cup of colored greens
1 cup of apples
5 carrots

34- Red Zone Juice

2 cups of apples
1/2 cup of beets
1 teaspoon of squeezed lemon

35- Blueberry Chocolate Reward

1 cup of blueberries
¼ cup of dark chocolate

36- Blue-nana Cocktail

1 cup of blueberries
1 cup of bananas
1 cup of soy or almond milk

37- Fruity Evening Cocktail

2 cups of apples
1 cup of oranges
1 cup of cranberries

38- Red Sunset

1 cup of cantaloupe
1 cup of papaya
1 cup of pomegranate

39- Avocado Avalanche

1 cup of soy or almond milk
1 cup of avocado
1 cup of apples

40- Tomato Soupy Juice

1 cup of soy or almond milk
1 cup of tomatoes

41 – Blueberry Addiction Juice

1 cup of plain yogurt
1 cup of blueberries

42- Creamy Fruit Juice

1 cup of plain yogurt
1 cup of bananas
1 cup of blueberries

43-Berry Tasty

1 cup strawberries
1 cup blueberries
½ cup of cranberries

44- Fast Track Juice

1 cup of apples
1 cup of oranges

45- Sweat Cream Cocktail

1 cup of soy or almond milk
1 cup of papaya
1 cup of apples

46- Orange Green Tea

1 cup of prepared green tea
1 cup of oranges

47- Chocolate Wish

1 cup of pomegranate juice
1 cup of yogurt
½ cup of dark chocolate

48- Heavy Delight

1 cup of oatmeal (cooked or uncooked)
1 cup of soy or almond milk
1 cup of bananas
½ cup of dark chocolate

49- Mello Dreams

1 cup of plain yogurt
1 cup of oranges
1 cup of cantaloupe
1 cup of papaya

50- Avocado Milk Delight

1 cup of soy or almond milk
1 cup of avocado

51- Red Bananas Cocktail

1 cup of bananas
1 cup of pomegranate juice

52- Strawberry Twist

1 cup of oranges
1 cup of strawberries

53- Orange Chocolate Juice

1 cup of oranges
½ cup of dark chocolate

54- Cran-apple Milk

1 cup of soy or almond milk
1 cup of apples
1 cup of cranberries

55- Tropical Treat

1 cup of soy or almond milk
1 cup of cantaloupe
1 cup of papaya
1 cup of apples

56- Zesty Orange Juice

3 cups of oranges
½ cup of beets
2 carrots

57- Apple Pie Milk

3 cups of apples
1 cup of soy or almond milk
½ teaspoon of cinnamon

58- Spiced Orange Tornado

4 cups of oranges
1 cup of papaya
½ teaspoon of cinnamon
½ teaspoon of ground cloves

59- Creamy Blueberries

1 cup of plain yogurt
1 cup of blueberries
1 banana

60- Zesty Fruit Juice

1 cup of apples
1 cup of oranges
2 celery stalks
1 teaspoon of lemon or lime juice

61- Tomato Hurricane

2 cups of tomatoes
2 stalks of celery
3 Carrots
1 cup of spinach
½ teaspoon of chopped parsley
¼ teaspoon of pepper

62- Tart and Delicious

4 carrots
2 cups of apples
2 cups of oranges
2 teaspoons of lemon or lime juice

63- Sweet Papaya Treat

2 cups of papaya
1 cup of soy or almond milk
¼ cup of dark chocolate

64- Cinnamon-Apple Oatmeal Juice

4 cups of apples
¾ cups of oatmeal
1 cup of soy or almond milk
1 teaspoon of cinnamon

65- Fruit Stand Special

1 cup of strawberries
1 cup of oranges
1 cup of apples

66- Peaceful Dream

1 cup of apples
1 cup of oranges
½ cup of pomegranate juice
1 teaspoon of lemon juice

67- Apple Tea Juice

1 cup of prepared green or black tea
2 cups of apples

68- Blueberry Surprise

1 cup of blueberries
½ teaspoon of lemon juice
½ cup of pomegranate juice

69- Tart Apple Juice

1 cup of apples
1 cup of spinach
1 teaspoon of lemon or lime juice

70- Spicy Fruit Juice

2 cups of apples
½ cup of oranges
½ cup of cranberries
1 teaspoon of cinnamon
1 Tablespoon of ground ginger
¼ teaspoon of nutmeg (optional)

71- Purple Delight

5 cups of apples
1 stalk of celery
¼ head of red cabbage
1 lemon or lime

72- Red Surprise

4 cups of apples
4 carrots
2 cups of Oranges
1 cup of beets
½ cup of spinach
One teaspoon of turmeric

73- Smooth Red Bliss

1 cup of apples
1 cup of strawberries
3 carrots
¼ head of red cabbage

74- Sensational Sensation

1 cup of apples
4 carrots
1 cup of beets

75- Delicious Concoction

2 cups of apples
1 cup of spinach
¼ cup of fresh parsley

76- Creamy Bananas

2 cups of bananas
1 cup of soy or almond milk
¼ cup of dark chocolate

77- Heavenly Juice Treat

2 cups of bananas
½ cup of pomegranate juice

78- Tea with a Punch

1 cup of prepared green or black tea
½ cup of pomegranate juice
1 cup of apples

79- Chocolate Banana-blueberry Fiesta Juice

1 cup of plain yogurt
1 cup of bananas
¼ cup of dark chocolate
½ cup of blueberries

80- Herbal Secret Juice

3 cup of tomatoes
1 cup of spinach
1 cup of broccoli
¼ teaspoon of black pepper
¼ teaspoon of minced ginger
¼ teaspoon of oregano
¼ teaspoon of thyme
¼ teaspoon of sage

81- Sweet Storm

2 cups of apples
1 cup of oatmeal
½ cup of pomegranate juice
½ teaspoon of cinnamon

82- Oatmeal Twist

2 cups of bananas
1 cup of oatmeal
½ cup of pomegranate juice

83- Spices of Life

4 cups of oranges
1 carrot
½ cup of oatmeal
½ teaspoon of ground cloves
½ teaspoon of cinnamon

84- Berry Surprise

1 cup of oatmeal
1 cup of blueberries
1 cup of strawberries
1 cup of soy or almond milk

85- Chocolate Cream Juice

1 cup of oatmeal
½ cup of dark chocolate
1 cup of soy or almond milk
¼ teaspoon of cinnamon

86- Unexpected Flavors

1 cup of cantaloupe
1 cup of papaya
1 cup of apples
1/4/teaspoon of cinnamon

87- Spiked Tea

3 cups of apples
1 cup of strawberries
1 cup of prepared green or black tca
½ of a lemon or lime

88- Dose of Happiness

4 cups of apples
2 cups of beets
4 carrots
2 cups of oranges
1 cup of sweet potatoes
1/2 teaspoon of cinnamon

89- Gentle Breeze Cocktail

2 cups of apples
1 ½ cups of oranges
½ cup of cranberries
½ of a lime
½ teaspoon of minced ginger

90- Sweet and Healthy

2 cups of apples
3 celery stalks
½ teaspoon of cinnamon

91- Tangy Orange Treat

2 cups of oranges
4 carrots
1 teaspoon of ground ginger

92- Smooth Sailing

2 cups of apples
1 ½ cups of carrots
3 stalks of celery
½ of a Lemon
¼ teaspoon of ginger
¼ teaspoon of turmeric

93- Spring Fever

5 carrots
2 cups of apples
½ cup of blueberries

94- Mello Meadows

6 carrots
2 cups of apples
1 cup of oranges
1 cup of sweet potatoes
1 cup of beets
½ teaspoon of ginger
1 teaspoon of Olive oil

95- Devilish Treat

1 cup of blueberries
1 cup of strawberries
½ cup of cranberries
1 cup of plain yogurt
½ cup of oatmeal

96- Holiday of Flavor

2 cups of oranges
2 cups of apples
1 cup of sweet potatoes
½ cups of almonds

97- Strawberry-Nut Sensation

1 cup of strawberries
½ cup of oatmeal
½ cup of soy or almond milk
½ cup of nuts (almonds, walnuts, pecans, hazelnuts, pistachios, or peanuts)

98- Heart Healthy Bloody Mary

4 carrots
1 cup of beets
1 cup of sweet potatoes

99- Hearty Heart Juice

3 cups of apples
1 cup of fresh parsley
1 cup of spinach
2 stalks of celery
½ teaspoon of ground ginger
1 lime

100- Red Surprise

2 cups of apples
1 cucumber
1 cup of beets
½ cup of fresh parsley

101- Dreamy Vacation

2 cups of apples
1 head of romaine lettuce
1 lemon

Conclusion

Thank you for purchasing this book! I hope you enjoyed drinking all of the recipes from this book and that you will share them with your friends and family.

I hope you'll find time to leave a review of this book on Amazon.com. Your comments are welcome and greatly appreciate

www.ingramcontent.com/pod-product-compliance
Lightning Source LLC
Chambersburg PA
CBHW070838290526
45795CB00002B/903